Weight-loss

(A story on how I lost 40kg)

By

Elizabeth Spencer

Disclaimer

Table of Content

CHAPTERS

Introduction

As soon as I dropped 25 kg, I contacted my thin pals, wrote emails, and exclaimed, "AH!!!!" I mean, becoming slimmer felt so amazing that I didn't understand why they weren't preaching the gospel of "slimness" all day, every day. Without visiting the gym or hiring a personal trainer, I dropped weight. I had no prior experience and had no idea what to eat or avoid. I was only trying to be good. As a result, I experimented on myself and made a ton of mistakes. I'll be discussing my journey from 110 pounds to 70 pounds in this book. Unfiltered. I'll discuss my battle with denial, my battle with food addiction, my wake-up call, my battle with consistency, and my battle with rice! All of my triumphs, struggles, and experiences. By the time you reach the last page, nothing about your life will be the same. My word is good.

Chapter 1

The Wake-Up Call

If you've read my blog, you'll know from the interviews I've conducted with people who have lost a lot of weight that we all have that moment when we are certain beyond a shadow of a doubt that we are overweight and that we need to make a change.

She could no longer put up with Nate's mother crying every time she saw her go to sleep because of concern that Nate wouldn't wake up after losing 75 kg. Ashley's experience was struggling to breathe while ascending a flight of stairs. If climbing "regular" stairs left her gasping for air, she must have realized she was in serious trouble. When Jasmine could no longer put on her garments, that was the turning point.

My mother's complaints had no effect on me. I also shied away from locations that required stair climbing. Why trouble myself, I asked myself. The fact that my clothes didn't fit only concerned me for a short while, and I decided to buy bigger garments instead of girdling myself. I kept telling myself things were not as horrible as they seemed, and I had more than enough people giving me what I wanted to hear around me:

You are only chubby; you are not fat.

You are simply big-boned.

You are beautiful the way you are, why are you trying to lose weight when I'm dying to gain weight?"

"You'll know you're not fat if you see a (genuine) fat person," the speaker said.

Geez! On a poor day, all I had to do was hit replay in my head to get things back on track. When I saw a large person, I was the kind of girl who would immediately communicate her disapproval to herself or to whomever she was with at the time. "Wow! Oh, that person is obese! Oh my goodness, I don't want to be like that. I only said that around individuals who would be quick to reassure me, so trust me on that. But as the saying goes, one day you'll realize that a thief lives to steal! it was eventually in 2013. I went shopping with a person who knew me somewhat well and had known me long enough to be aware of a problem (as if being fat was not bad enough). Here are the things he kept saying to me as we exited the vehicle and entered the parking lot:

Are you able to see that woman, Sara? That's how chubby you are.

Look over there, you are heavier than that woman.

Observe that lady? You dress that way.

"Like a duck, that's how you walk."

"You look like that."

Sara, you look overweight, and it makes me uncomfortable to be around you. Many people have never succeeded in getting me to be entirely silent during such an attack, but those who know me well have. But this particular day, I was really shocked. These were the types of folks I would typically look down upon and feel like a model in comparison to. These were the types of individuals I condemned and felt bad for. I realized all of a sudden that these folks were just like myself, if not better. I had been wholly denigrating. Confusion was all I could feel at the time. It turned into fury as I reached home, still feeling disoriented. However, this is the first time as I Many people have never succeeded in getting me to be entirely silent during such an attack, but those who know me well have. But this particular day, I was really shocked. These were the types of folks I would typically view with disdain, feeling like a model next to them.

gaining weight, you are not in shape. "Stop eating so much; you're not hungry."

But none of the soothing remarks had any effect. The ear plugs fell that fateful day as a result. I started to question why I hadn't heard this before after this encounter. Did those around me not show me enough care? Was it too hard to talk to me? The most likely scenario is that I was repeatedly warned in subtle ways, and I completely disregarded them. Alternatively, I may have been so skilled at projecting happiness that everyone thought "Sara is just fine." Everyone else can see when you're in denial, but you can't, and most of the time, those around you feel Simply said, keeping quiet about it is safer so that nobody has to face the repercussions. Such remarks are taken seriously by obese persons. You are not healthy. Stop overeating; you are not hungry. But All the soothing words had gone unheard. The ear plugs fell that fateful day as a result. I became too difficult to talk to after this event. When people around you feel it is just safer not to tell you that you are fat and you are wondering why they don't tell you, it is important to understand that telling anyone that they are overweight is challenging because the speaker knows that what they are saying is not something that will please the recipient. Was I told several times in different subtle ways, and I completely disregarded it. The speaker is aware. Because it is beyond of his or her control how the information is interpreted, and that it is highly likely that such a statement will have an adverse effect on the connection.

Therefore, I had to put myself in their shoes before I got angry with everyone who had allowed me to eat my life away. I also came to the realization that it is more challenging when a thin person is advising a large person on weight loss. Oh my, the advisor's reply would have been in the past.

"How dare you criticize me?"

Do you know the tale I tell?

Are you aware of how I got here?

The difficulties I have encountered?

Do you realize that the only reason I would have the audacity to ask such questions is because I am well aware that the "never been obese, slim person" cannot adequately respond to any of them, and I cannot afford to be teased?

If someone told you that you looked good (and were obese), two things were going on.

Do not be duped, my dear friend. Be aware of what you are hearing before getting excited if you have been informed that you are big and lovely. Nobody, not even being overweight, can take away from you your magnificent creation. But to say that you are attractive while overweight is false. Stop fooling yourself that being who you are makes you happy. Stop describing You simply have huge bones or are overweight. Stop referring to oneself as gorgeous and bold and stop using hashtags.

You cannot claim to feel good when entering a store with a high degree of certainty that you won't find your size or when you are led to the maternity section because you are larger than the items in the XL section. You cannot claim to be content with your arms becoming nearly the size of your thighs. When a tailor says, "Madam, this cloth will not be adequate for you," you cannot claim that you are happy. You cannot claim that you have never wished that you were smaller so that you could wear particular clothing.

You can keep convincing yourself that being overweight makes you feel good, but honey, I don't buy it.

Which do you think the people in your life would prefer—a smaller you or a fatter you—if given the option?

What version of me would you prefer if you asked your family, your coworkers, or even your boss? Really, do you think they'll say, "Oh, I want you to be obese?"

Being overweight indicates any one, all, or more of the following:

"Your body is not within your control."

"You are powerless over your thoughts".

"You lack self-control."

"You can't refuse temporary satisfaction."

"The denial you exhibit"

"You are a slacker (even if you are a successful CEO).

(If you're big, you're lazy.) You don't care about yourself enough to change.

Additionally, your forehead is inscribed with all of these things. Nobody except you can see it. Before you get upset with me because the com attendants started to avoid me. Please don't berate me for telling you something you don't often hear. The "denial zone" needs to give way to the "healthiest and greatest you there can ever be zone," not because I said so, but because you deserve to live a long and healthy life.

Homework

1. Do you think you are overweight? If the truth be told, the answer is yes, then take a big breath and relax.

2. Recognize and accept

3. Verify your BMI (BMI). It is a straightforward weight-for-height index that is frequently used to categorize underweight people based on their height in meters (kg/m2). Check if you are as thin as you believe! If you are aware of your weight but unsure of how much, check! Your BMI will provide you a clear picture of your situation. Many folks don't even know the smallest thing. However, their BMI indicates that they are overweight compared to their

height and weight. Know your status by checking your BMI.

Chapter 2

Wait! What the hell brought me here?

Some of you just tested your BMI and were shocked by the results. You can probably now imagine how I felt when my BMI revealed that I was an Obesity Type 1 person. As if being overweight wasn't horrible enough, I had also earned the designation of Obese Type 1. It is crucial that you complete the homework before moving on to the next chapter before I continue. Only if you carefully read through each chapter of this book will you get the most value out of it.

The fact that I was overweight really ached! My cheeks started to tear up. I sobbed and cried! "Sara, how on earth did you get here?" I then asked myself. How did I get to be this terrible size? How did I move unnoticeably from M to L to XXL? You must ask yourself the same question if you are overweight. Don't say what most of us would say, please. I don't like salads, I eat late, and I like swallow to swallow. You are not obese for that reason. So you ate those, and now you are fat! However, that is not the main cause. You should honestly consider why you eat the way that you do, without any restrictions. The majority of my life, I was large. I've never been skinny for very long, and when I was, it wasn't on purpose.

However, when I was 11 years old, I was chubby and had high blood pressure. My parents encouraged me to participate in all sports; I played soccer, tennis, and even caddied for my father when he played golf. Because my brothers had male friends with whom we could play, it was beneficial.

Do not imagine that I suddenly became interested in all these outdoor sports and decided I wanted to be slender at the age of 11. That was definitely not the case! The doctor took great pains to frighten me to death. If I continued living the way I was, he warned, I might pass away at any time. A child doesn't want to learn about death. He informed me that I had to stop eating Pringles! For me, that was a significant event. I was therefore driven to shed weight, and I maintained my health until I was fifteen. I then lost my father.

All of a sudden, food was my sole solace, and I continued to use it as a pacifier for all of my troubles going forward. everything from minor annoyances like being frustrated by traffic jams to breakups and even headaches! As eating progressively turned into a habit, then an addiction, I felt compelled to eat even when I wasn't hungry or having any problems. It seemed that if my mouth wasn't moving continually, I wouldn't be alright. I increased my weight. My health suffered, which ultimately hurt my self-esteem. Who can thrive without a healthy sense of self? And who is overweight and has a solid, positive self-image? I made several attempts to lose weight, but they were all mental. Every day, I vowed to start the following day, but every morning I found a reason to put it off. When I did manage to overcome myself, I would fast occasionally or diet for a few days (I looked forward to the church announcing fasts, for me it was not about the spiritual journey but an opportunity to lose a few kilograms). I would experience a little period of success before returning to square one and occasionally adding a little additional a few weeks later. When you deal with the fruits instead of not, that is what happens. the main problems. I kept putting my attention on healthy diet and exercise instead of dealing with the most crucial issue—my mentality! I had to be honest with myself and admit that I was overweight, that I had a food addiction, and that if I didn't address the underlying issue, dieting and exercise would be pointless. I could only think of a more modern solution to my difficulties after that. It became simpler to lose weight and maintain a small figure—not easy, but simpler. It was undoubtedly challenging. It is difficult to break any habit or overcome an addiction, but it becomes simpler to control if you have a better understanding of who you are and what drives you. I found that questioning every thought was one thing that truly helped me. For instance, if I were out to dinner with friends and everyone was ordering steak and fries, and I was feeling particularly puckish, I would pause and ask myself:

Why do you want a steak, exactly?

"Because everybody is placing orders?

"Who cares if everyone is placing an order?

"I feel like I wouldn't be eating as much as they would be," she said.

"What is pleasure?

eating something that will make you feel bad and cancels your four hours of work?"

"Won't I feel a lot better about eating when I reach my goal? By the time I accomplish my goal, will this supper be finished on Earth?

When I had finished posing these queries to myself, I would discover that I had ordered a healthy dinner, felt good about it, and had resisted the urge to consume whatever the other diners were having. I wasn't any longer a victim of my emotions. I had to deal with the issue of pacifier use while eating.

Every time I encountered a struggle and felt the urge to eat, I would ask myself, "Are you upset? Hell yes!"

"Why…?"

"Because…"

"What are the benefits of eating?"

"Please cheer me up."

"How much time?"

"Briefly."

"How would you feel following a meal?"

"Bad."

"So you will have to deal with the additional eating guilt in addition to the previous challenge?"

"Yes."

What more can you do right now that will enable you to overcome the difficulty?

"Reading about it and observing how others handle it, or speaking with someone who has handled this."

(There are always more advanced ways of handling everything, from dealing with a challenging employer to overcoming allergies.)

"I still feel hungry."

Instead of cake and ice cream, I'll just have water and carrots.

"Deal."

This is a typical scene from my inner dialogue. It's been a huge assistance to me. It took some time for me to get into the habit of pausing and considering my motives; prior to that, I would ask the questions without waiting for an answer. I would merely consume food. But once you get going, pausing and asking questions becomes quicker and easier until ultimately it becomes automatic.

Prior to addressing the underlying reason of your current situation, postpone any weight loss efforts. Today, ask yourself, "How the heck did I get here?"

Homework

1. Consider your route to this location. Write down the event or events that occurred, and then consider your sentiments and the reasons behind them. You'll find that it's actually not a problem when you honestly ask and respond to those questions; rather, you are just experiencing what I refer to as "uninvestigated ideas." Just picture me gaining weight because my father passed away. He was now at peace, sleeping soundly, and sending his baby girl his best wishes. Meanwhile, I was still living through his funeral almost 15 years later, using that one experience to ruin the rest of my life. What event or events, then, do you still hold dear? What recollection from yesterday are you bringing into the present? Do it in writing!

2. Think about your future plans for handling these problems. Make sure that, whatever you decide, it

improves your self-esteem. Will learning new facts improve your mood? Read!

Does exercise improve your mood? Exercise! Does meditation aid? healthy eating? Remember to pay attention to how you feel; you might not be happy about it. Sadly, some of us develop an addiction to feeling sorry for ourselves, so when we do something that makes us feel good, we find a way to sabotage that. The good news is that we have it within us to overcome any obstacles we may encounter.

Chapter 3

Emotional vs Physical conflicts

By being honest with yourself about how you got to where you are, hopefully you have established a progressive approach to handling your current circumstance. Additionally, you can start to see that gaining weight or being obese is an emotional issue rather than a physical one. You aren't overweight because you can't be thin; rather, you are fat because you won't be thin. You aren't losing weight because you can't, but rather because you haven't made up your mind to. A professional swimmer who had gained over 80kg caught my eye. When I read that she was once a professional swimmer, I was curious because she is someone who is not afraid to work out and has discipline. She was a pro. She didn't gain weight because she lost her swimming ability; rather, she did so because of unsolved mental concerns. When you observe the lives of those who have successfully lost weight and kept it off, you can tell that there was a time when they could hardly move from one place to another without running out of breath; now, they can run 5 kilometers without stopping, and they carry on with their daily activities as if nothing has changed. You must be wondering how they underwent the shift and what was different. If it is the same person, has the same body, and has not altered, then the only thing that has changed is the way they think and how they have chosen to view themselves. I was only able to perform five skips in 2013.

Even the 10 was difficult, to be honest. To catch my breath, I would lean over and grab my knee. I was unable to maintain my balance long enough to even plank. I sobbed! I can't even perform the most basic forms of exercise; how can I possibly hope to reduce weight? I didn't want to feel like an even bigger failure for failing to lose weight because I already felt like a failure for allowing myself to become so obese. I would host a pity party and lament how I would always be obese (thinking about it now, I must have looked pathetic). However, I was simply too exhausted to remain where I was and felt that I had to do action, so I looked for inspiration. I searched for before and after pictures of Jennifer Hudson and Monique, telling myself that these women didn't have two heads. I would push myself every day, and before I knew it, I was performing 100, 200, 500, and now 4,000 skips. I used to hold a plank position for three seconds, then five, ten, and now two minutes. What altered? my thoughts Where you want to be will continue to appear impossible until you are sick of where you are. You have to really want it. Nobody could possibly have a strong enough desire for you to reduce weight.

I have to confess how thrilled I am when someone contacts me by phone, email, or in person and requests, "Please tell me how you did it! I'm willing to try anything. I've received emails that have brought me to tears. I am constantly willing to share since I am aware of how much this experience has transformed my life. You need to observe how their demeanor changes after receiving my response. Typically, their reactions are, "Ah! Oh, and I also can't stop eating swallow and rice, and I also can't stop eating chocolates! Exercise? Can't I just follow a simple diet? I wish I could take a photo of myself and present it to you. People anticipate that I'll have one medication they may take and that they'll then go to sleep and awaken 40 kg lighter. Obviously, there isn't! Losing weight will take time, just like you didn't just wake up fat; it took time. Put an end to looking for a quick remedy. If you began improving yourself as soon as you realized you were overweight you would have lost considerable weight by now already, but you were too busy complaining it demanded too much. Not to worry, I am also guilty. In fact, it is because of the guilt that I don't get mad at the responses I get from people, because it reminds me of same things I use to say. I really believed I could lose weight as easily as I gained it, by eating what I wanted. Romantic right? Somehow I was so special that the law of seed time and harvest didn't apply to me, that I could still eat all I wanted and lose weight, it didn't take long for me to realize it was better to accept the truth and get to it than dance around playing chess with my life.

Most of us want the outcome, but we also want to skip the steps necessary to get there. The time has truly arrived for you to put an end to your justifications. It's time to quit claiming that you cannot afford a personal trainer, a gym membership, or pricey diets. You can be sure I didn't require any of those. Without a trainer, I performed all of my exercises alone at home, and my diet was inexpensive. I found out a lot and saved a lot of money.

Homework

Ask yourself

1. How much do I desire it?

2. What am I prepared to renounce to obtain it?

My darling, if you are aware that you are not prepared to renounce your old life in favor of the new, then you are not. Old behavior doesn't produce fresh results for anyone.

Chapter 4

Dear Journal

The few who had the guts to tell me that I was eating too much must have become weary of debating me. I believed that although I consumed food exactly like everyone else, my body responded in a unique way. But as I made efforts to become more self-aware, I decided it would be a good idea to start keeping a food journal to track what, when, and how much I was consuming.

This ostensibly simple idea was trickier than I had anticipated. I found it challenging to always record every single thing I ate. I often found myself purposefully leaving out some foods and failing to provide complete descriptions of my meals because I was embarrassed to be eating again and recording it, so I tried to limit my intake. I would include the rice and chicken but leave out the entire box of cookies and two Snickers bars. Without specifying whether it was a glass or the entire pack, I would write juice. How practical, yes?

After that, I would regretfully refuse to eat since I did not want to add two more bowls to my meal. You may image how I felt when I realized I was lying just to myself. After wasting paper for a week, I made the decision to do a strict and frank self-evaluation. After a typical day, my journal looked like this:

Day 1
2 large mugs of chocolate beverage, each containing 2 sugar cubes for a total of 4 cubes.
5 tablespoons of milk and 2 squares of chocolate - 8am
8 a.m.: 4 slices of yam, egg sauce, and sausages.
10am, half a pack of TUC
1 bag of plantain chips at 11:00
11 a.m. Coke can
Chicken pie: 12:00
A LOT of rice, chicken, and plantains around two o'clock
Ice tea, half a pack, about 2:00 PM
8 p.m.: rice, beans, and meat
Bread with peanut butter at eleven o'clock
4 sweets throughout the day
A can of coke at one in the morning

In a single day! After the first week, just picture the horror. I would never want my adversaries to find out about it. I would write this before that:

"Egg and yam"
"chicken with rice"
"beans with rice"
I would put that in writing and let everyone who cared know that I don't eat as much as they "see" know.

I didn't drink any water, so don't believe I forgot to add it. Since juice, beverages, and cola all include water, I could go days without even thinking about the existence of water. It sounds like you?

At the conclusion of the first week, I entered my room, locked the door, and read each line. I sobbed, but I sobbed! like someone had passed away. I was puzzled as to how I managed to eat so much without even realizing it. I felt incredibly, really ashamed by myself. Then I understood that my body wasn't reacting differently to what I was eating like everyone else, but rather that what I was eating was reflecting in leaps and bounds. I was committing suicide.

Homework

So think twice before telling yourself you don't eat as much as you do. For one week, keep a thorough journal and then go over everything. I encourage you to eat as you normally would because there is a strong temptation for you to skip meals only to be able to grin at your diary at the end of the day. The need for the truth. Additionally, I advise writing down your thoughts as soon as you eat because you are more likely to forget or leave something out if you wait until the end of the day. You can do it on a writing pad or on your phone.

Chapter 5

A Vision Board

You must be wondering what a vision board has to do with anything at this point. People's faces express one thing when I bring up this topic: "We want to reduce weight!! Please skip to the section where I'm told what to eat, what not to eat, and how to exercise. I also remind them that, rather than the other way around, they came to me to learn how I did it. I lost weight over the course of ten months, spending five of those months gaining and losing weight as a result of ignoring the most crucial factor—my thinking. If the mind does not undergo an orientation program, all of your life's endeavors will be in vain.

I just didn't understand how it was possible to lose weight and then gain it back—this is difficult and uncomfortable. Gaining the weight back is discouraging because losing it is no walk in the park. I just knew that I had had it with self-pity.

I maintain a vision board. Now, it has transformed into a vision room. I display images of the tasks, destinations, and possessions I hope to complete. It has succeeded. I update it occasionally, removing my accomplishments and adding new objectives. So I questioned why I hadn't posted anything on weight loss. I continued to gain 70 kg. I chuckled. Even though I was afraid that someone would pass by my vision board and make fun of me for wanting to lose 70 kg, I still looked through magazines to find images of thin people that I aspired to look like and hung them up. It was crucial for me to include the image of the woman running and the nutritious meals so I could constantly remind myself that exercise and a balanced diet were necessary if I wanted to achieve my objective. I posted a calendar with smaller targets so that the overall aim wouldn't seem so overwhelming because it looked practically impossible. I also uploaded before and after pictures of Jennifer Hudson. On my PC, phones, and other devices, I used it as my wall paper and screen saver. I questioned myself, "What can I do right now to move me closer to my goal?" every day as I gazed at my walls. My vision board served as a daily reminder and helped me put things into perspective. It's unimaginable. the emotions I experienced at reaching 70 kg and the tears that streamed down my cheeks as I stared at my wall. Wow, I succeeded.

Homework

1. Get a picture of your ideal figure, the precise amount you want to weigh, and images of people exercising, then post it everywhere. You can post it on your refrigerator to serve as a reminder to pause before choosing to eat mindlessly. Don't include words like "don't, can't, fear," etc. on your board. Employ verbs like can, do, and will. Play around with images to create a mental map of your destination.

Chapter 6

Pay Close Attention to Details

Like I mentioned in the chapter before, I discovered images of ladies exercising. I also received a platter of wholesome food, after which I made a calendar. I set a goal for myself to drop 1 kg per week, and each week I would mark it off when I achieved it. Making sure you come up with realistic approaches to achieve the goals is a crucial step when using a vision board. If you don't write them down somewhere, you could become demotivated rather than inspired. If you have ambitious fitness objectives, you could feel a little overwhelmed after finishing your work. How will I drop 50 kg, you'll be asking yourself? 40kg? 30kg? 15kg….? 5kg?

Considering that 5 kg is only It doesn't get any simpler to complete with just one number. The mentality required to lose 5kg is the same as that required to lose 50kg. When people inquire about my weight loss, I respond that I didn't begin with the intention of losing 40 kg. I first believed that the maximum weight I could reduce was 5 kg. I couldn't even exercise for ten minutes without feeling like I was going to pass out, so how on earth could reducing 40kg be even remotely possible?

After much trial and error, I realized that if I kept concentrating on losing 40 kg, I would always feel overwhelmed. As a result, I created a calendar of smaller goals. I gave up worrying about my weight. I was concentrating on the minor details instead of what I was unable to do at the time. Just concentrate on losing 1 kg, I kept saying. Just concentrate on executing 100 skips and holding a plank position for 10 seconds. I stopped stressing that it would take me 30 minutes to do 100 skips or a one-minute plank. I nonetheless done it! I set a goal in my calendar to lose 1 kg every week, and I actually did it. The more times I crossed off my success, the more driven I became. I started losing more weight as a result of my increased exercise, accelerated pace, and ongoing challenge. When I used to stare at 40 kg, plank for 5 seconds, then collapse to the ground, I would think to myself, "Sara, how would you lose 40 kg when you can't even keep yourself up for just 5 seconds?" It didn't feel like that anymore. "Sara, you can now do 5 seconds, remember you couldn't do 3?" I began to explain. You have a long way to go before you lose 1 kg. The ability to motivate oneself is crucial because there will be times when you look to the walls for encouragement but they won't provide it to you because they can't, even if they wanted to. You must learn how to continually inspire and motivate yourself. When things are difficult, take a glance at your vision board, but keep your attention on the details.

Homework

1. Create a calendar with little objectives that add up to your main objective. Make a plan, including the precise actions you must take to achieve your goals, and then carry it out.

Chapter 7

Modifying One's Palette

Near my home, I discovered this pretty amazing business where you can buy pills to expand your palate. Buy the "like vegetable pill" if you want to start appreciating your vegetables, and in an hour you will consume all the vegetables you can find. WISH ME WELL! There is no such thing, honey!

I'll let you peek inside my gorgeous mouth, and you'll see that I don't have any cavities. I had no holes to fill by the time I was 16 since they had all already been filled. Except for those that cannot be filled, I don't have any unfilled teeth. As you can see, I detested going to the dentist since it was torment, but it didn't stop me from loving sweets. I was a sweet mouth; I didn't have a sweet tooth. Imagine me planning to lose weight...the things that went through my mind. I found it revolting to put anything in my mouth that didn't have sugar or taste sweet.

I had to stop doing everything I like and had grown accustomed to because I wanted to reduce weight! Yes! It served as sufficient justification. I questioned what I would be eating because it may be quite challenging to please someone with a mouth like mine. I used to be the kind of person who would only eat the chicken and rice, ignoring the salads. I would gulp it and drink lots of water as soon as I could if I were in a situation where I had to behave so I wouldn't have to deal with it. I am aware that changing diets can be difficult on its own. Once I had a People inquire, "So what do you now eat?" after seeing a list of all the foods I quit eating. They gave the impression that rice was the only option for food.

And it's funny how when individuals email me about joining the Total Makeover Program, they provide a list of the foods they don't eat so I can make accommodations. You can't learn anything new if you stick to your old routines.

How can I learn to eat these things is the actual query. The response? Perfectionism is attained via practice. I had to try several things before I discovered how to enjoy the salads; I didn't just start loving them right away. At first, I began combining it with eggs daily; three salads per day equaled three to five eggs per day. day, only to learn that having that much was unhealthy. When I read that removing the yolk made eggs healthier, I declared, "I'm not taking out the yolk; what is the point of having an incomplete egg?" I therefore had to stop using the salad dressings, hmm! Okay, so I started experimenting and eventually found that the best way to enjoy my dish was to make it colorful and cut the vegetables into really small pieces, so that I could consume them fast and move on. I decided to relax and added some spunk with spices like black and white pepper. In fact, I would take my time eating my salads, especially if I would stop drinking water as I grew weary. Now that I know how to appreciate salads, I use this method to enjoy all the healthy foods I once believed I would never like. Now, I even relish cooking and eating such meals. It takes some time, I can assure you, but the key is to have a good attitude. Finding out about each ingredient's nutritional value and the benefits it was contributing also helped me. If I ate something and it didn't feel right in my mouth, I would tell myself, "It's good for your eyes girl, eat!" The most intriguing part is that after achieving my physical goal, I stopped eating healthy and began having extramarital affairs with my ex-boyfriend and ex-girlfriend. A soft drink, chocolate, and ice cream. By the next morning, I felt sick. I was extremely constipated and thought my body had been polluted. I was in awe. How is it that my body detected an alien in my system so quickly? The same things that my body had formerly become accustomed to were suddenly foreign. I had to detox to regain my sense of wellness, but that doesn't mean I no longer eat those things. Instead, I only occasionally do so now, and when I do, I only eat a small amount—often just a bite or two. I've learnt to pay attention when my body signals that it's had enough. Pause and pay attention to your body rather than your habit—that is crucial.

Homework

1. Choose a healthy meal that you currently detest (but that you are not allergic to or are being told not to eat by a doctor). It could be salad or seafood. Work your way up to it until you find it appetizing enough to eat. Is it just your thinking, the presentation, or the seasoning? Train your taste buds to discover new ways to appreciate food, eat carefully, and feel and taste each and every mouthful. You'll find that it's not quite as horrible as you thought.

Chapter 8

Resisting Temptation

When you decide to take this journey, you will face many temptations that you must resist. I'll discuss my struggles and the obstacles I had to conquer in the hopes that it would be helpful. I had to push through myself. Nothing else or anyone else was the issue—I was. I had to learn to ignore all the nice-looking items in the grocery store and continue walking. I would hope that my favorite cookie could fly into my basket without my touching it so that I wouldn't have to feel bad about eating it, but instead, I would stop and think about all the calories I would add and how many hours of exercise it would require to burn them off. I would sigh and turn away, burning it. However, I made a list of everything I was going to buy and took the exact amount I needed before the chance to lose on the mental battlefield presented itself. I avoided the wicked aisles totally, and I didn't bring anything home that I wasn't going to consume (if it is in your house, in your fridge, you will eat it). It was simple for me to exercise control because I live alone. But if I went home to visit my family, it was a very other story! I was surrounded by individuals who had no concern for their health. I had to prepare food for a group of fat-loving individuals. calories and carbohydrates. However, I prevailed and made my food separately. In order to avoid being tempted to eat because I was too exhausted to make my own supper later, I took sure to avoid waiting until I was actually hungry before starting to cook. They all made fun of me, I assure you. I was instructed to put my diet on hold for just one day so that I could enjoy myself with them, but I didn't, and after a few weeks of continuous work from my mother, she was able to.a team member who shed 10 kg. Now that my mother was looking up to me, I was unable to turn around.

Everybody enjoys nice things. Everyone desires to lead a healthy lifestyle, yet the majority of us only require encouragement. My family joined in because of my results. I prepared one wholesome supper for us, which helped to reduce my tension. But one thing was crucial— before I exposed myself to it, I had developed the ability to conquer the challenge on my own. I was far from anything or anyone who may induce me to give in. Few people will get the chance. It's difficult to resist peer pressure, yet resisting temptation is one of the keys to maintaining consistency.

my initial advice is that The expense should always be considered. Most individuals desire to go without adequately planning first, and you know what they say about planning. You are intending to fail if you don't make a plan. This also applies to losing weight. People just wake up and declare that they are beginning their journey for the hundredth time, but they are unaware that failure to account for the costs was one of the numerous reasons it failed in the past. You won't see fresh results from your old habits, I'll repeat it. You must be prepared to do something you have never done if you want to experience something you have never experienced. which also includes waking up an hour earlier than you do so you can work out, even if that is 4am. It includes convincing your husband to change date nights to work-out nights. It includes reducing the number of weddings you attend because when you do, the tray of small chops disappear quickly. It means that instead of watching five movies on Tuesday (because it is only a thousand naira with free soft drink and popcorn) you watch just one or none.

To see a movie at home, you might have to get inventive and buy data to download it instead of renting it. Though it may sound simple, you will quickly learn that cutting yourself off from the people and things you love and are accustomed to, even if they hurt you, is incredibly challenging. This means that you will need to separate yourself from things and people that do not support your current goals and are not assisting you in achieving them. During moments like this, you begin to comprehend people's struggles and the reasons why they continue to engage in abusive and parasitic relationships, drug use, and other behaviors despite knowing they deserve better and that they may not survive.

It is crucial to assess your "savings" to determine whether you have enough money to cover the cost. It is not enough to simply calculate the cost. You must determine whether you require a "loan." Since you don't want to become a forgotten project. Ask your partner for assistance if you are married. Have an honest discussion with yourself. Inform them of your struggle and solicit their assistance. Tell your buddies you won't be having sleepovers any longer since you need to commit to a plan and would value their support. Talk to your family and let them know you need them to keep an eye on you and prevent you from eating certain things at specific times. and not jeer at you or put you down.

Homework

1. List the five do-able actions you'll take right away to help you resist temptation. You must be completely sincere. Should you quit going to weddings, please? Do you need to ask the woman who brings lunch to your workplace to cease delivering a portion for you even though you're feeling bad? Note it down and keep in mind that you just need to give up that one thing until you achieve your objective.

Chapter 9

Consistency/ Resilience

I want to let you know that you are a weight loss failure if you have repeatedly tried to lose weight with little to no results. However, I want you to know that being chilly is not necessarily a bad thing before you get upset with me for being so cold. Every person who has ever started this road and succeeded attempted and failed to lose weight several times. Multiple failures have the advantage of teaching you numerous ways not to do something.

For instance, even if you attempted clean eating and exercise and it was successful, two months later you are back to your old habits and are now overweight. You should be aware that approach won't work. However, a lot of us want to have our cake and eat it too. You want to eat when you want, how you want, and expect to receive the results you want... Now that you know, The proverb "to repeatedly do the same thing in the same way and expect a different outcome" is one that we have all heard. I can't stress enough how crucial consistency is. The single thing that likely distinguishes individuals who eventually lose weight from those who don't is this. Those who lose weight are not always smarter or stronger on the physical level than those who do not. The only distinction is that those who succeed choose to press on regardless of the suffering, discomfort, still-steady weight, unfitting clothes, and other setbacks; they just keep going!

I frequently receive emails from people who describe their attempts to lose weight and how they gave up after a while. These emails make me smile because the solution can be found even in their confusion. I wonder if they ever consider the possibility of continuing. They show a great deal of fear. "Are you sure I can ever lose weight?" is one phrase I frequently hear. Are you certain that I will benefit from this? It almost sounds as though they have no control over their lives at all, that they have no idea where they will be tomorrow, and that their lives are at the mercy of the wind. As you read this, wherever you are right now, is a direct outcome of all the choices you made or didn't make. Start now to work toward where you want to be this time next year. Focus on the details, create a vision board, and most importantly, keep moving forward, as I previously stated. If you want to, you can make it. Until you find yourself unable to lift your leg the morning after exercise, you could believe you want it badly enough. It sounds like you?

This gets me to my second point: consider the price. Do you ever set off on a trip without first figuring out the expense of getting there? Do you begin constructing a home without first determining the project's cost? You shouldn't do this to avoid having a project abandoned halfway through. Most individuals get fired up and delighted about the prospect of losing weight and fitting into a gorgeous dress for a birthday or wedding, but they often forget that they also need to adjust their lifestyle and persist until they see the desired results.

Homework

1. Add up the price. Determine how many hours, days, weeks, or months you'll need to achieve your original and long-term objectives.

2. Determine the cost to you in terms of money, time, events, parties, etc.

3. Make a plan for how you're going to behave consistently this time. What requirements must be met?

Accountability?
group of friends?

Chapter 10

Individuality

Now that we have reached the final chapter of this lovely book, you must be asking why there isn't a handbook outlining the exercises you should perform and those you should avoid. It's easy to understand why. We are all unique, and the sooner you start accepting that, the more quickly you will advance. I can assure you that everyone is extremely different after seeing my metamorphosis and the transformation of the 40 men and women who have completed my program. Because they utilize a one-size-fits-all strategy, most people fail on this path for a variety of reasons. "Sara tried this and she dropped so much weight," and "Linda did that and it worked," are common statements. Don't you understand? Sara or Linda are not you; you are you! You are not Sara or Linda; you are living your own life and competing in your own race. The client I spoke with was trying to reach her goal by eating healthily and exercising, but she was continually feeling ill. After careful research and planning, we discovered that she was sensitive to practically all of the nutritious foods on her meal plan. Listen, it's risky to get sidetracked by other people's travels; pay attention to your own so you don't have an accident. Some people will lose weight that is visible on the scale after eating salad for one day, while others may not lose visible weight but will shed dress sizes after consuming smoothies for a week. The majority of us experience overload because we tend to concentrate on others' journeys rather than our own.

But the elements I stressed in the earlier chapters are the ones that need to be taken into account before what you eat or don't consume.

Accept the circumstances as they are. Recognize that you are overweight rather than "large boned," since there is no such thing. People have hefty, dense bones, but this is not the same as being overweight. Even though you are as light as a feather, you might weigh a lot.

Consider the price, be willing to make some sacrifices, realize that it will be challenging, and give up trying to have your cake and eat it, too. Create the habit of being independent, self-reliant, and motivated. There will be times when you will need the support of family and friends, but they will be preoccupied with taking care of themselves.

Realize that one of the reasons you are still overweight is not that you are physically weaker than those of us who have lost weight; rather, it is because we continued to work toward our goals while you gave up. Know this: There will be times when you'll look in the mirror and wonder how your enormous hanging stomach can ever get smaller. At those times, keep in mind that your success is determined not by the size of your enormous stomach but rather by the size of your will.

Accept accountability for your deeds. Don't put the blame for your situation on anything or anyone. Now is the moment to make changes if you do not like where your choices have led you. You are overweight because you choose to eat after losing your job, not because you lost it. Own your errors and grow from them. Keep in mind that after you achieve your goal, all the food you enjoy will still be available.

Please remember this if you take nothing else away from this book. No matter how bad things appear, EVERYONE can change, and the only thing getting in the way of your development is you. So, here is your last assignment:

Homework

    1. Get out of your own way, first!